M000011868

SEX
and the
SINGLE
GIRL

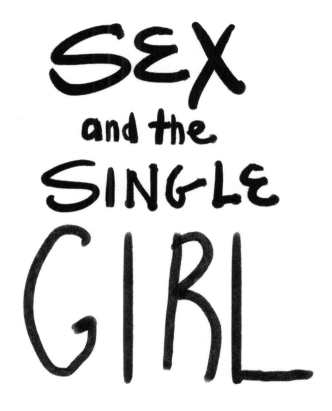

SEX
and the
SINGLE
GIRL

A [SLIGHTLY OLDER] GIRL'S GUIDE TO
DOMINATING THE DATING WORLD

Written by Anne Grey

Illustrated by Leah Roszkowski

Copyright © 2016 by Anne Grey

All rights reserved. No part of this book may be used or reproduced in any manner whatsoever without prior written consent of the publisher except in the case of brief quotations embodied in critical articles and reviews.

The methods described within this eBook are the author's personal thoughts. They are not intended to be a definitive set of instructions for your own life, nor legal advice. You may discover there are other methods and materials to accomplish the same end result. Some names and identifying details have been changed to protect the privacy of individuals.

For more information contact:

Anne Grey

www.annegrey.com

Printed in the United States of America

ISBN Paperback: 978-0-692-63737-1
ISBN eBook: 978-0-692-63738-8
Library of Congress Control Number: 2016902077

Cover Design: Leah Roszkowski
Interior Design: Ghislain Viau

Table of Contents

Introduction   1

1 We Don't Want to Have Your Babies and
       We Don't Want Your Money   · 5

2 You   19

3 How to "Order In" a Man   31

4 Keep It Safe. Keep It Smart. Keep It Sexy!   45

5 Now Is Your Time   57

6 We Are Made of Stars   67

Conclusion   71

The Single Girl's Guide to Resources   73

Bibliography   81

Acknowledgments   85

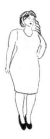

Introduction

I wrote this book with single women in their late thirties, forties, and fifties in mind. I believe this midlife age can be a time of change, a time to reevaluate, and a time to fully embrace life. Personally, I didn't have a choice when my marriage of eleven years ended. I had no option other than to reexamine my life and how I wanted to live moving forward (other than drinking profusely and crawling under the covers, which I did do for a time!). Whatever your situation, I believe this age for a woman can be incredibly powerful.

I also think a lot of changes are happening in the United States in terms of attitudes about sex, sexuality, gender, and the roles of men and women. Gay marriage is now legal. Trans-sexuality is becoming more accepted. The millennial generation (whose parents were part of the original free-love movement) is much freer with their sexuality and getting married later in life. On top of all of this, the world is becoming much smaller, greatly enabled by technology and ease of travel, so the sexual openness of our European friends is slowly influencing our more traditionally conservative thinking.

The most obvious changes in all of our lives are the incredible advancements in technology. We're always connected now, which can be good and bad: bad in that it's sometimes difficult to disconnect from work and achieve some semblance of work/life balance, and good in that technology is brilliant at enabling human connections, many of which would not have been possible otherwise. From dating apps to Facebook to Snapchat to FaceTime to easily accessible porn to remote-controlled sex toys, the world has become a smaller place and, in my opinion, a much more exciting place.

As my journey as a newly single woman of forty-four evolved over the last year, my curiosity led me to explore my sexuality. I did tons of reading, took a class or two, and met some lovely young men along the way. It hasn't been perfect. I've made some mistakes along the way. But overall, it's been fantastic. I am truly living life. I feel more alive than I have ever felt before, and I'm ready to tell the world all about it!

It's worth noting that though my adventures have been with younger men, the overall message of owning and embracing your own sexuality—*regardless* of the age of men you choose—is the point. I chose younger men as a place to start. You should start with whomever you want.

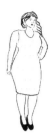

Chapter 1

We Don't Want to Have Your Babies and We Don't Want Your Money

I t all started on Thanksgiving Day 2014. The prior week, my then-husband and I agreed that our marriage was over, and he moved out. Happy holidays. Ugh.

I was fortunate enough to spend Thanksgiving Day surrounded by a group of wonderful friends, the majority of whom were fabulous gay men. As the wine started flowing, I divulged my newly separated status to the group and was met with more wine and fantastic support, of course. As dinner moved toward pumpkin pie, I asked my friend Sean if I should get on Tinder (a dating app that I knew he was familiar with). Without hesitation, he exclaimed, *"Yas, gurl,* get back on that horse! Get out there! Where's your phone?"

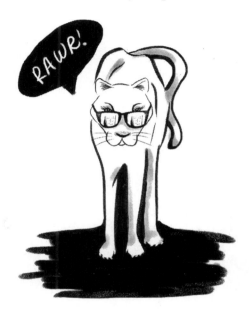

I had already downloaded the Tinder app, but was a bit scared to use it. Sean immediately took my phone, opened the app, started swiping, *and* started communicating with my matches. I was awestruck, and my amazement only grew when I saw he was only picking super-young, super-hot guys (of course he was)—and they were matches for *me!* What was happening here?

Within forty-eight hours of digesting turkey, and after texting and a bit of sexting (more on that later!), I found myself hightailing it in a taxi to Bucktown to meet up with Michael, a twenty-eight-year-old consultant with a six-pack and an adorable face. He was an all-American frat-boy type—the kind of boy I would have died for in my twenties. Now I was forty-three, and here he was in front of me.

It was a Saturday, in the middle of the day, broad daylight, and I was nervous and excited. I hadn't had sex in quite some time, and it was time to break that pattern. I brought along a bottle of red wine to help calm my nerves. We drank the wine, we laughed, we flirted—and then we spent the afternoon in bed. He was kind and generous and fun. I couldn't help but wonder every five minutes—was this *my* life?

So began my exploration of younger men. Everyone knows Mrs. Robinson, but I don't think I believed this phenomenon of younger men being hot for older women was real until I experienced it myself. And younger men were all about me!

Even as I kept going on dates with these younger men, I couldn't quite believe it. Finally, I was so curious that I just started asking my dates: "Are you always attracted to mature women?" The answer, consistently, was "yes." A large group of younger men that I knew personally felt that older women are the absolute most sexy, goddess-like creatures on Earth. And my life was about to get a lot more interesting!

I think journalist Frank Kaiser expresses the truths about mature women perfectly:

As I grow in age, I value older women most of all. Here are just a few reasons . . . to sing praises of older women:

An older woman will never wake you in the middle of the night and ask, "What are you thinking?" An older woman doesn't care what you think.

An older woman knows herself well enough to be assured in who she is, what she is, what she wants, and from whom. By the age of fifty, few women are wishy-washy. About anything.

. . . Her libido's stronger.

Her fear of pregnancy gone.

Her appreciation of experienced lovemaking is honed and reciprocal.

And she's lived long enough to know how to please a man in ways her daughter could never dream of. (Young men, you have something to look forward to!)

. . . An older, single woman usually has had her fill of "meaningful relationships" and "commitment." Can't relate? Can't commit? She could care less. The last thing she needs in her life is another dopey, clingy, whiny, dependent lover!

. . . For all those men who say, "Why buy the cow when you can get the milk for free?," here's an update for you. Nowadays, 80 percent of women are against marriage. Why? Because women realize it's not worth buying an entire pig just to get a little sausage! (Kaiser 2000)

Kaiser is funny, and more importantly, he's right: The combination of older women and younger men makes a lot on sense on several different levels. At this point in most of our lives, we are indeed financially stable, independent, past our childbearing years, and we've lived enough life to know who we are, how we want to be treated, and what we want. We've loved and lost, traveled the world, and have racked up a fair amount of life experience. For many of us, we've already been married (and divorced). Another legal commitment is just *not* likely something we are seeking. Our bodies might not be as tight as they were in our twenties, but the confidence we've gained over the years more than makes up for it.

We offer younger men wisdom, stability, confidence, beauty, intelligence, and experience that they are not finding in women their own age. Conversely, I find that as a newly single older woman, I seek much of what younger men have to offer: no children, no ex, nothing complicated, the thrill of young ambition, general physical fitness, and a *very* healthy libido.

The Science of It All

I distinctly remember one of the very first evenings I shared with Jack, an extremely stressed-out twenty-eight-year-old law student. We met up at a bar and had a couple drinks. He was wildly ambitious and hardworking, and he wasn't looking for a serious relationship. Neither was I. After we slept together, I was thinking about going home—and to my surprise and delight, he said, "Oh, hold on for a few minutes, and I'll be ready to go again." This was a phenomenon I hadn't thought about in years! Younger men can go for multiple rounds, and so can older women. Our sex drives line up perfectly. And with Jack, it wasn't just one more time . . . it was *two!*

I got home exhausted and, of course, still curious. I'd had no idea that I was that sexually hungry. It turns out, though, that there's a biological explanation for my sex drive: My body thinks that this is my last chance to reproduce. So, even though I've already chosen to not have a child, my biology is driving me hard to procreate. The other thing to take into account is that for most women, sex is more psychological than physiological. As we get older, we're more comfortable with ourselves, and our confidence—sexual and otherwise—allows us to know what we want in bed, ask for it, and get it.

The University of Texas at Austin did an interesting study recently about the high sex drives of older women. I found it particularly compelling because it wasn't based on science, but on an online questionnaire that was sent out to 827 women in three different age groups. Apparently, the lower our fertility level is (and the older we get), the more we think about sex, fantasize about sex, and seek sex. Sounds about right!

I had discovered from personal experience that biologically, older women and younger men do align. We brilliantly align. And the more I thought about it, the more I wanted to know about younger men and their drive as well. According to Ava Cadell, PhD, a Los Angeles sexologist and founder of LoveologyUniversity.com, men produce the most testosterone around age eighteen (UTNews 2010), but it takes a full ten years after the peak of production to reach maximum testosterone levels in the body. Basically, my new fling with twenty-eight-year-old Jack was right on target. This was making more sense by the minute.

Bridging the Generation Gap

I came of age in the 1980s. Ronald Reagan was president, America was ultraconservative, and my parents were still registered Republicans (I'm proud to say that now, my eighty-four-year-old mom campaigns for Hillary. Go, Mom!). I also happened to have grown up in a small Iowa town with a population of about six thousand. All of this is to say, the word "conservative" really didn't begin to describe my upbringing.

The expectation for a girl like me was to get married, have babies, stay in that town (or at least nearby), and live happily ever after. Well, I didn't quite follow the rules. I didn't get married until I was thirty-two. Even then, I intentionally didn't procreate. And I escaped to urban life during college, never again to return to small-town existence.

I'll never forget a conversation I had with a little old lady from my church back home. Upon visiting the church on one vacation, I proudly presented my fiancé to her. Her reaction? "I thought I'd be dead by the time you got married!" After that, it seemed like every time I was home, everyone in town was curious about when we were having a "little one." And then, when I got divorced, well, . . . I must be just a huge disappointment to all those folks.

Sex was also not a topic that was discussed. Ever. I remember meeting my first gay friend when I was in high school. I also remember wondering how all that fit in with the Bible. I even went and talked to my small-town pastor about it. He kindly told me that it was OK if I had a gay friend, and God loves everyone, but participating in any gay acts was wrong according to Jesus and the Bible. And it wasn't just gay sex that was a sin; most sexual acts or even thoughts were just plain bad—or at least that's what I learned to believe. Even though a lot of us did experiment with various forms of sex, there was an underlying shame associated with it. You didn't want to get a "reputation" for being a "slut."

In adulthood, I lived in Sweden for a couple years, and I discovered that the cultural perspective on sex across the pond is completely different. I remember being a bit shocked that Swedish parents let their kids have their teenage girlfriends or boyfriends stay overnight. Sleepovers between significant others were completely normal and accepted. But the more I thought about it, the more sense it made. Sex isn't shameful or bad. The European mindset would have been a much healthier way to grow up.

So there's me—us—and then there are the millennials. They were raised by baby boomers, who were themselves the start of the sexual revolution in the '60s. That revolution, of course, meant **evo**lution, and fittingly, a study went up in the 2015 Archives of Sexual Behavior called "Changes in American Adults' Sexual Behaviors and Attitudes, 1972–2012." (Twenge 2015) Pretty straightforward, right?

"The changes are primarily due to generation—suggesting people develop their sexual attitudes while they are young," said study leader Jean Twenge for an article in the Los Angeles Times. (Kaplan 2015) Having grown up with those baby boomer parents with a freer attitude about sex has led this generation of millennials to be quite open in terms of sexuality, and it just keeps getting better with time.

That openness is making its way deeper and deeper into our culture. I ran across the most incredible article about a disposable, instant STI test that a company is trying to bring to market (I found it in Forbes Magazine, of all places).

(Frezza 2013) The takeaway was that millennials are the perfect generation to market this product to because sex is often *recreation* for this group. Commitment-free fun for all could be even better if they were able to instantly test their partner for STIs. Millennials don't seem to have this sense of shame—or, for that matter, modesty—when it comes to sex.

I think millennials are a little lucky. They've been born into a more open environment for exploring sexuality, whereas our generation grew up often thinking sex was dirty and shameful. At some point, though, most of us have worked our way out of the shame by our late thirties, forties, and fifties. And if we find ourselves single at this point in our lives—hooray for us! We can own our sexuality, enjoy our bodies, and even learn a thing or two from a lovely young man or ten. As older women have lived through and escaped their conservative upbringings, younger men simply view sex as fun. And even through we are more mature in years, millennial men can push and challenge us as we think about and further embrace our sexuality.

A Little Feminism for You

I have never thought of myself as a feminist. The word "feminist" often comes with a lot of stigma. People think "feminist," and then they think "activist," for better or for worse. It's the kind of activism, too, that seems to be borne out of necessity: When things are blatantly imbalanced between the sexes, the feminists show up for justice!

The pursuit and acceptance of a "traditional" relationship—one where the man makes more money, has more power, and is the stronger figure in the relationship—came hand in hand with my conservative upbringing, as did other distinctly non-feminist-sounding values. The thing is, though, that I never had antifeminist values in my upbringing. Both my parents worked. Both my parents took charge. Both of my parents, well, *parented*. It's only occurred to me just recently that this kind of equality itself is feminism.

So I was fortunate and I didn't know it. That, of course, changes as you get older, and now that I'm recently single, the subject has become more relevant and interesting. I've been inhaling Helen Gurley Brown and Betty Friedan and Gloria Steinem and seeing how all of it fits into my life, and it's simple! Steinem, who, when asked why she never married (Steinem 2015), replied, "I can't mate in captivity." Having just ended an eleven-year marriage, I found this statement to be the funniest and most profound at the same time.

Furthermore, there's now a whole other interesting area to explore called "sex-positive feminism," which is completely new to me, but worthy of my time both now and in the future. The premise is that sexual freedom is core to women's freedom. It's been around since the eighties (ironic, right, Ronald Reagan?), but seems to be gaining more traction—perhaps because of the generational shift that's coming into play.

15

I have only just begun my interest in and study of feminism, but I know something even bigger is happening in society. We are in the middle of a major paradigm shift. As an older single woman, I make my own money. I am free. I have the power to choose what I want, when I want it. I can realize most any aspiration and shape my own path. Now is an incredible time to be an older woman.

This shift has created a change in consciousness, according to Dr. Noam Shpancer. In his article "The Cougar Conundrum," (Shpancer 2012) he points out that the rise of the older woman/younger man relationship celebrates the beauty of the aging woman and her active role and power in society. That's right. Modern women can go after what we want. And we can get it. Especially if it's a younger man!

Tales from Tinder: Liam

Chelsea, a good friend of mine, met twenty-four-year-old Liam while she was on vacation in London. They actually connected online in advance, and even had some FaceTime dates to get to know each other before she flew out to visit. She and Liam talked about everything, from her recent divorce to safe sex to favorite positions.

When she got to London, Chelsea wasn't quite sure what to expect, but Liam was there at baggage claim, waiting for her. He'd planned an amazing evening for them, including grabbing beer at one of his favorite pubs, dinner at a Korean barbecue joint, and cocktails at a hot spot in Soho. The evening was filled with flirtations and fun . . . and they had an even better time in her hotel room that evening!

Chelsea tells me she still hears from Liam about once a week via WhatsApp, and they have FaceTime dates when they can make it work. Last I heard, they were also exploring a vibrator that he could control remotely from across the pond!

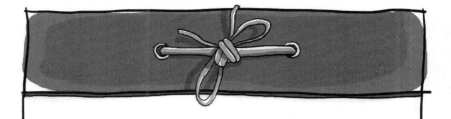

→ Now is an incredible time to be an older woman, as with financial independence comes freedom, and with freedom comes the power to choose what we want, when we want it.

→ Highly advanced dating apps are providing today's women with a tremendous number of avenues to enhance their self-esteem, social connectivity, and sex lives.

→ Younger men have much to offer older single women, and many of them are supremely eager to be presented with the opportunity!

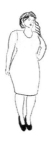

Chapter 2

You

You Are Beautiful

I am a size twelve on a good day—a *very* good day, when I've already abstained from carbohydrates for a few weeks and tortured myself with spinning classes on a regular basis! Throughout most of my adult life, like so many of us, I've wanted to be thinner, and have consumed myself with various plans to achieve the body I thought I needed. I've done the low-carb diet, Weight Watchers, the five-hundred-calorie/day two-days-a-week diet, and I did actually manage to follow the Master Cleanse for ten days without fainting—not a small feat! I've put myself through *all* of this to end up more or less the same size, year after year. Society truly does impose an unattainable ideal of a woman's body upon us, and it's very difficult to not get sucked into believing this is the way we're supposed to look. The end result, of course, is that we struggle every day.

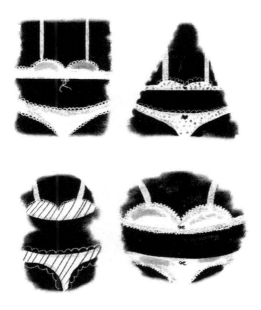

Granted, I had been on the "divorce diet" when I started meeting younger men, so I was about fifteen pounds lighter than I usually am. All the same, the reaction of the men was nothing less than amazing. These younger men *adored* my voluptuous body! I am seriously Rubenesque, and now I've never felt more sexy or wanted, because guess what? Men. Love. Curves.

They love big boobs. They love a big ass (thanks, Kardashians!). They love a real woman's body. Young, hot, sexually liberated men think we curvy girls are where it's at. According to the 2015 SKYN® Condoms Millennial Sex Survey (SKYN 2015), 46 percent of millennial men like big boobs and 44 percent like big butts. I'm betting that number is even a bit higher.

Another thing that younger men love is the confidence of an older woman. According to psychotherapist Jane Polden[1], women simply have fewer insecurities by the time they reach middle age. I can feel the difference between Pre-Marriage-Single-Twenty-Something Anne and Post-Marriage-Single-Forty-Something Anne, and I *love* it. It's a great, big, palatable difference. I was so consumed with what others thought when I was in my twenties. Those were really tough years in regard to self-esteem and body image, and I remember being outright relieved when I turned thirty. No amount of money would convince me to live through my twenties again—and every woman I know past her twenties has said the same thing. Those years were awful. I used to get on the scale every single day and beat myself up when I was up a mere pound or two. I'd feel terrible about myself until I could take those pounds off. I let the scale rule my self-confidence, and, frankly, my happiness.

Now. I know I'm no supermodel (and a good twenty pounds heavier than I was in those years), but I generally don't worry

1 http://www.brisbanetimes.com.au/news/life-and-style/sex-and-the-older-woman/2009/02/22/1235237423253.html

about the way I look. In fact, I feel quite sexy and confident most of the time. Of course, I still have days where I don't feel my best. A couple days ago, I felt like a sausage stuffed into my "Not Your Daughter's Jeans" casing. I've put on a few pounds recently, and I was feeling it.

The difference now, though, is that I don't let it get to me. It doesn't stop me from feeling sexy and good about myself.

That evening, I met up with my friend Nick (aged twenty-nine) who took one look at me and said, "God, I love your body." And just like that—I felt even sexier.

My intention is not to dismiss any feelings that any of us have about our imperfect bodies. I understand the struggle is real for all women everywhere, including myself. But life is short. Most of us are in the second half of our lives. It's time to embrace and accept our bodies as they are. Right now. If you feel like you're not confident in the way that I'm describing, now is the time to find ways to embrace your body and your sexuality. Men aren't perfect either. No one is. We all have insecurities. We are all human.

So here are a few fun confidence-boosting tips from my personal archive. Use them! Remember, this isn't about getting you a man for a night; this is about being happy about yourself, with yourself. These tips aren't a magic wand, but they'll get you going!

1. **Move!** I walk a minimum of ten thousand steps a day. If I don't walk, I go to the gym and walk on the treadmill

or spend some time on the elliptical machine. And while walking, I listen to really fun, current pop music to keep my spirits and my heart rate elevated. Spotify has great curated playlists. My favorite is "TGIF." I crank that up and move my ass!

2. **Try something new**—every day, if possible! Eat at a new restaurant, listen to a new podcast, watch a new movie or documentary, learn a new word (or study a new language!), meet a new person—perhaps a new man. If you're constantly opening your mind to and learning new things, you really start to feel alive and in tune with the living world around you.

3. **Make sure you are surrounding yourself with positive, like-minded, confident people**. This one is a little tough, but sometimes we don't realize that some of the people we hang out with are really bringing us down. Motivational speaker Jim Rohn famously stated that we are the average of the five people we spend the most time with. This is kind of a scary concept if you really think about it, but let it motivate you to think about whom you hang out with and whom you let into your life.

You Are Sexual

I have one more fun tip: **Have sex!** By now, you have (mostly) accepted your body and are feeling more confident, so now's your chance to try it all out. Sex is great for so many reasons (as we know!), and one of them is that you literally feel better about yourself after an orgasm. According to researcher Gemma O'Brien, during orgasm, we experience a "diminution of self-awareness" and "alterations in bodily perception." (Webb 2011) In other words, self-consciousness just drifts away, leaving us with a more positive body image in general. That's right! The more sex we have, the sexier we feel. It's a great cycle that we can keep boosting if we so choose.

I'm pleased to tell you that it gets even better. According to the same study, having sex and meditating lead to the same result: They shut off the noise in our minds. Meditation activates the left side of our brain, while sex activates the right side. Both lead to allowing ourselves to center our thoughts—which then allows us to return to the rest of our lives filled with more creative and productive energy. Stopping the noise can also lead us to a state of altered or higher-consciousness—bliss, in fact! Who knew that something so incredibly pleasurable could also be balancing from an energy standpoint? Mediate, schmediate.

We already know there is a biological need to have sex. But the chemical response is even *more* fascinating. When we have an orgasm, we release dopamine, which increases strength and confidence, motivation, well-being, and healthy bonding. We're then consumed by a rush of oxytocin, which not only reduces cortisol (a stress hormone), but also makes us feel stronger bonds with our partner and with the world in general. Oxytocin offers a bevy of wonderful benefits: It enhances the feeling of being calm and connected, increases our curiosity, facilitates learning, heals, repairs and restores, lowers blood pressure, and protects against heart disease. (Last 2015) Sex feels fantastic, *and* it's healthy! How awesome is that?

You Are Human

After my divorce, sex was initially about healing. It was my first impulse when my husband and I called it quits. I sought sex without understanding the meaning, and it was OK. Thanks to my friends, I was in a cab within days, headed to have sex with a complete stranger! It was intuitive. It felt good. It was validating. It was powerful. But what I didn't understand was that it truly was *healing*. Sex is one of the very most primal ways humans can express and heal ourselves. It resets our systems in a way that nothing else can.

As Wendy Strgar, founder and CEO of Good Clean Love, writes: "After we eat, drink, and sleep, the next thing we are is sexual. Reawakening to our capacity to feel happens when we stop paying attention with our thinking minds and focus instead on our sensory capacity. Besides the most obvious reasons to invite and cultivate a pleasure response of how good it feels, there are hundreds of medical studies that reinforce the multilayered impact of a healthy sexual response to every other aspect of our wellbeing." (Strgar 2015)

I couldn't agree more with Wendy. When we find ourselves in a situation where we have shut down our feelings (such as a bad marriage), sex can be one of the best ways to start experiencing life again.

As I continued to dig into the humanness of sex, I remembered Maslow's hierarchy of needs (at least I remember *something* from high school!). It is most often portrayed in the visualization of a pyramid, with the most basic of human needs at the bottom. Maslow calls this bottom tier the "physiological level," and it includes air, food, drink, shelter, warmth, sex, and sleep. These are all absolutely required for survival as a human being. Physiological needs are thought to be the most important; they should be met first. There you have it. As humans, we have needs. To connect with another human in the act of sex is a need. A real need. Nothing is more intimate. Nothing is more powerful. Nothing is more human.

When thinking about the humanness of sex, one story from well before I was married, comes to mind. On 9/11/01, I was living in Chicago, watching the second plane hit the Twin Towers live on *The Today Show*. I remember walking to work with one eye on where I was going and one eye on the Sears Tower. After everyone was sent home from work, I went home to my little studio apartment on the fourteenth floor. I had nonstop CNN on my TV, and so I had a direct view, again, of the Sears Tower. It seemed like everyone in Chicago had abandoned the downtown area and that I was alone in the world. I have never felt more isolated and scared.

The following weekend, I went to visit my mom in Iowa. She mentioned that an old classmate of mine had asked about me and that he'd like to see me when I came home. This guy was cool, but not at all my type. I met up with him anyway.

We ended up seeing each other quite a lot over the next few months. It turned out to be a lovely affair, but one that never would have occurred had 9/11 never happened. The relationship didn't make any sense, but at the time, it was a huge escape from my urban existence.

I wish that mind-blowing sex was as easy as stripping and connecting your parts, but in my experience, I've found that you really do need to *genuinely* like the person with whom you're going to get naked. This is the tricky—and often most elusive—part. This type of connection doesn't necessarily happen the first time you meet someone, and in some cases, it may never happen. You have to be willing to meet up with quite a few men, and you need to be vulnerable enough to open yourself up to the possibility of a connection in order to find a relationship that is going to be sexually fulfilling. I've found that the best kind of sex can be transformative and energizing, but it also requires a trusted partner—one who lets you truly be free in expressing your sexuality. This is the type of relationship you need to be seeking. And with a younger man, all of this is possible. And gratifying. And lovely.

Tales from Tinder: Jeff

Jeff and I connected fairly early on in my Tinder explorations. He was twenty-six—a little young for me—but adorable, with a mustache, a beard, and a twinkle in his eye. Plus, he was a teacher, and I figured that at the very least, I'd get a good conversation out of him!

I reached out, and we got to texting almost immediately. There were a lot of hot texts about 50 Shades of Grey-type of activities (which I had recently read), so expectations for something mind-blowing were fairly high. But when we finally met, that 50 Shades energy just wasn't there. It was OK, sure, but not fantastic. I'm fairly certain Jeff was a bit intimidated by me, and he was never as comfortable around me as I would've liked.

The fun part of this relationship, though, is that over the course of months, he always stayed in touch. He sent me flirty Snapchats and notes full of wit and silliness. And during the darkest days of my divorce, Jeff was always there with a quick snap of his handsome face and a message that brought a smile to my face. We are still good friends to this day!

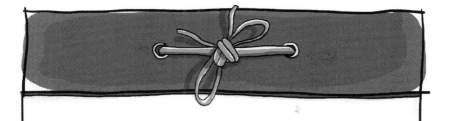

➜ Stop stressing over the size of your butt and trying to emulate a Barbie doll, because it's finally been scientifically proven: Men **LOVE** curves!

➜ Raising the level of your self-confidence is the most constructive thing you can do to enhance your beauty.

➜ Sex is a true, legitimate human need, and one of the very best ways to heal ourselves, emotionally speaking.

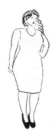

Chapter 3

How to
"Order In" a Man

For ages, men have been in control of choosing women. You know it and I know it. At private, Playboy-type clubs, in harems, in arranged marriages—men have had the power to choose the exact kind of woman they desire. They've always had the power.

Well, guess what?

We women now own this power in our smartphones. We can choose exactly what we want, when we want it. Most interestingly, this shift was predicted long ago by engineer, physicist, and futurist Nikola Tesla. He actually predicted that wireless technology would empower women, forever changing society's gender roles. (Popova 2015)

After I had been on Tinder for a month or two, I remember going over to a friend's apartment for a holiday party. She's young and pretty open-minded, so I told her and her friends that I was having the time of my life, meeting younger men online. I remember saying that meeting younger men was as easy as ordering takeout. I could literally meet up with a gorgeous young man as easily as I could order a pizza. I am not kidding, even one bit; it's that easy. And I invite you to give it a try!

Ever since the Thanksgiving episode, Tinder has been my app of choice. Initially, it was because after just separating from my husband, I definitely wasn't interested in anything serious, or even the possibility of something serious. C'mon, I had been married for eleven years—it was the time for uncommitted fun! And Tinder has the reputation of being the least serious of the online dating apps currently out there.

But beyond it being the most "casual" app around, Tinder's interface also makes it incredibly appealing. Here's how it works: You set your geographical boundary (Tinder is a geo-located app, so, for example, I have it set to only suggest men within a ten-mile radius of my location) and select the age range you desire. Magically, a ton of men pop up, as if in a deck of cards. You start looking through them and swipe

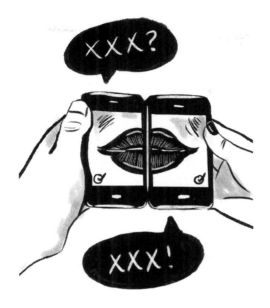

left (no, thanks) or right (yes, please!) mostly based on how attractive you feel they are. The beauty is that you can absolutely choose the hottest, youngest, most appealing guys that you want and they will never, ever, know if you choose them unless they choose you as well. It's brilliant. And shallow. But mostly brilliant. And it's how I truly discovered that younger men are attracted to older women. In fact, I initially had the lowest end of my age range set to twenty-seven. One day I was bored and lowered it to twenty-three . . . and my matches blew up! *Crazy.* I was fascinated.

Choose Your App. Or Apps.

As I mentioned, Tinder is my app of choice, though there are many others available (and likely more all the time!). As of July 2015, twenty-six million matches are made daily on Tinder. (Tinder 2015) The demographics of Tinder are also favorable, as 45 percent of Tinder users are ages twenty-five to thirty-four: exactly the age range of men I prefer.

First, you need to download the app and set up a profile. Some apps, like Tinder, have you connect to the app via Facebook. This scares a lot of people, but please don't worry. None of them post anything to your Facebook page without your permission, and your friends on Facebook will never know you signed up (not that it matters— as I discovered, tons of single people I know are already on Tinder!). The bonus here is that the app will tell you if any of your friends are connected to one of your matches.

Show 'Em What You Got

Now that you've chosen your app, it's time to set up a profile! And the very first step is to upload photos. (This is especially true of Tinder; it is, after all, about visuals.) Some apps will allow you to upload your photos directly from your computer or phone, and others, like Tinder, will ask you to connect with Facebook.

I recommend that the first picture be a very clear picture of your face. Mine is a selfie, but a good one! It shows me in an interesting space (Borough Market in London) and has a filter on it that makes me look like I'm glowing (goddess quality!).

The second picture I have is a professional work picture. Showing that you're professional can be helpful, especially if you're seeking professional men. And the third is a full-body picture. It's important to give men a realistic idea of your body type. Honestly, it'll make you much more confident when the time to meet rolls around, since he'll already know what your body looks like. It also takes away the need for them to ask (rudely, sometimes) for more pictures of your body.

My fourth pic is kind of sexy. It is a boob shot, if you will. In a tight football T-shirt. You don't have to do this one, but calling attention to your assets never hurts!

Make a Statement

After you upload your pictures, you'll see a place to say something about yourself. For the longest time, I left this space completely blank. And it didn't seem to matter. Depending on what app you're using, it might, but I was on Tinder. And the best part about it, for me, is that Tinder is all about if you are attracted to someone—physically. Or not. Period.

I recently populated that area with a few of my interests and a quote from Frida Kahlo about finding a "lover who looks at you as if you are magic" or some such crap. In the context of Tinder, I really think the description doesn't matter one bit (though I do read the description on men's profiles and I do judge them). Men just want to see if they find you attractive. That's the bottom line with an app—and a mission—like this!

Get Going

So now what? Your pics are uploaded, and you've crafted a description (or not). You start swiping. Now, if you're super picky like I am, you won't have very many right swipes. This was highly concerning to me at first, but soon I realized that I could be as picky as I wanted to be. The thrill of a "match" with a hot, young, sexy man would soon be mine! I seriously picked only the youngest, hottest, most desirable men, and nearly died when they were a "match." Be super selective. You're allowed to be.

Playing Hard to Get

When you "match"—as in, when you both swipe right, when there's mutual attraction—the app pops up and gives you the permission to start messaging with said match. Don't. You heard me. Don't.

Yes, I grew up in the era of "The Rules" (look 'em up: http://therulesbook.com/) and I followed them religiously. (A lot of good they did me, since I ended up getting divorced after I followed them all!) The Rules are rules for a reason: They've worked in the past! I do recommend that you wait for the man to reach out first. I think it's highly interesting—and telling—to see what men lead with. See what they have to say. Are they clever? Do they ask you a thought-provoking question? Do they say something that makes you laugh? Do they ask you out for dinner (keeper!) or start trying to sext with you? Or do they open with "DTF?" (DTF, for the uninitiated, means "down to fuck." I admit, I had to look that one up on Urban Dictionary. And, yes, some people are that rude.)

Yea or Nay?

At this point, it's your choice to decide if you want to respond. Another beauty of this app is the ability to "unmatch." If anything, at any time, doesn't feel good about corresponding with your match, you can stop it with the click of a button. No commitments here. No need to feel bad if it doesn't seem interesting or feel right to you!

These apps also have features to help you stand out if you really like someone. Tinder, for example, has a "Super Like" feature. You can Super Like one person per day, and the app will send that person a notification. It's helpful because then you don't have to match to understand that someone really wants to meet you. I haven't used this feature yet to select a man, but I have received several Super Like notifications. And—surprise—they have all been from men under the age of thirty.

After the Match

Sometimes, you'll start chatting and the conversation quickly turns to a sexting-type situation. This is fairly normal, from my experience. Often, men will ask you if you want to move to texting or WhatsApp or Snapchat.

This is where things get a bit complicated. To put this in context, according to a 2014 study by security software firm McAfee, nearly 50 percent of adults in the United States send or receive sexual content via video, photo, e-mail, or messaging. (American 2014) Clearly, sexting is becoming mainstream in our society, but you have to listen to your gut and do what's best for *you*. If you do decide to sext, it can be quite hot. It can even be useful; they see what they're getting, and so do you. Men are more than happy to send you "dick pics," even unsolicited!

If you live in the same area, though, I recommend pushing back. It's much better to meet in person, do a chemistry check, and see what's real. Remind them that they've already seen a realistic version of your body in the picture, and you will not disappoint!

Sexting 101

Sexting is a tricky subject, but like anything else, it can be mastered—and made *safe*. Here are some tips to get you going.

- If you take a picture of your naked or half-naked body, make sure your face is not in the picture!

- Snapchat is safer than texting or a WhatsApp exchange, as the pictures supposedly disappear (though nothing is guaranteed in our cyber world!)

- Use filters and lighting; they enhance your already-gorgeous body. Why not make it the best it can be? A quick tip for Instagram: Switch your phone to "airplane mode" so it won't post the picture. Then, take a sexy picture, put all the filters and awesomeness of Instagram around your picture, and "post." It will save in your photos but not actually post, and then you can upload and send it to a hopefully deserving young man!

- Don't send anything that you aren't comfortable sending. Understand that anything you send to anyone can end up in the public domain. Try to send anything super revealing only to someone you trust. Use your instincts. It's a strange, crazy new world!

Taking It to the Next Level

Real conversation often comes better to people than sexting, and if that's what you'd prefer, absolutely go for it! Remember, everything you do here is for you, and you're in control. Check out some of my tried-and-true conversation starters:

- If he doesn't disclose what he does for a living in his profile, ask. I realize you aren't looking for a husband, but you *are* looking for someone you can talk to. Good sex is highly enhanced by a connection beyond the physical. The way I see it, the more ways you can connect, the better!

- Ask for his last name so you can verify that he's not lying about said profession—or anything else—by checking him out on LinkedIn. If he has nothing to hide, then it won't be a problem. Plus, you can read all the nice things people have to say on their LinkedIn profile about working with him!

- If he doesn't have a LinkedIn profile, ask if he minds connecting via Facebook or Twitter or Instagram. Tinder actually allows you to connect your Instagram account to your Tinder profile. I don't recommend this because even if you are not a match, people can stalk you. That said, after you've matched, there is no harm in checking out his feed to get a better sense of who he is.

- Now that you know his first and last name and possibly where he works, Google them to find more information about them from the World Wide Web. *It's OK* to dig through his past.

- Ask if his pictures are recent. And if his Tinder profile doesn't have enough photos, ask for some more. There is usually a reason that someone doesn't have many pictures, like the fact that he/she gained about fifty pounds since the others were taken. So, while you have time, ask!

- Don't text for too long before actually meeting in person. I did this once and found myself unable to connect the flirty, fun text relationship I had with this man with the actual serious and slightly boring man sitting in front of me when we finally met. *#fail*

Crossing Borders

One of my favorite Tinder features is a paid option that allows you to "Tinder" in a different city. You can turn it off and on as you need it (other apps do have an equivalent feature). I used it on a couple different trips, and it worked really well. Connecting with a local always gives you a different and more authentic experience of the culture or country you are visiting. And, while I don't mind traveling alone, it's very nice to have a dinner date or two planned out in advance—not to mention the admiration of a young, foreign man.

It works the other way around, too. Lots of people—especially those who do a ton of travel for work—use one of these features, and I find it fun to connect with someone who's visiting. It's particularly exciting because you never know what you're going to get or what you might learn! Oftentimes, dinner at an elegant restaurant is involved . . . and usually a swanky hotel room (plus, hotel sex is hot!). This doesn't just apply to one-night stands, either; if someone travels to your location with relative frequency, you'll have a few fun rendezvous to look forward to!

I submit that meeting on an app like Tinder or online is much safer than meeting someone out at a bar. You can do all of this background investigation before you ever meet. And if something doesn't check out, or feel right—unmatch! Immediately! *You* make the decisions about whom you want to meet. *You* choose what you want based on initial texting and investigation. *You* are in control! Share your own story of a great date (or a dinner date gone wrong!!) with me at anne@ annegrey.com, and I'll post them on my website!

Tales from Tinder: *Rob*

My friend Amy swiped right on Rob, a consultant from the East Coast who happened to be in town on business. He had to head home before they met in person, but that didn't stop them. They ended up texting . . . then Snapchat texting . . . and then having phone sex for almost six months before they ever met in person.

I found it sort of strange that Rob was content with this kind of virtual relationship, but he was really into hot older women, and he swore that Amy was the most beautiful woman he'd ever "met." He loved that she could talk him to orgasm, and she loved how powerful she felt doing it—and they're still going at it today!

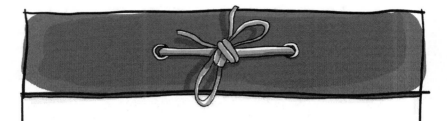

→ Today's woman possesses the power to find, select, and obtain the exact type of man she chooses, rather than simply hoping to fit a man's ideal, as was typically the case in decades past.

→ Tinder is an excellent, safe resource for older single women who are seeking to engage in no-strings-attached sexual relationships with hot younger men, but be sure to do your behind-the-scenes research on the men you choose to meet in person!

→ When creating your profile on a dating app, make sure to upload photos that show you in your best light. A flattering headshot, a professional photo, a full-body image, and a sexy shot should do the trick if you select them wisely!

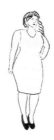

Chapter 4

Keep It Safe. Keep It Smart. Keep It Sexy!

After being married for years, safe sex wasn't something I had worried about in quite some time. I've never had to worry about unwanted pregnancy either; I decided years ago that I didn't want to have children, so I got sterilized. Now, though, I was single and on the prowl, and I knew it was time to brush up on my knowledge. There were STIs I didn't know about, preventative measures to take—and even sexual skills I probably didn't have after being with the same partner for so long, doing the same old thing.

I'll be honest. I needed some education. Fortunately, I was able to get started with my "higher education" pretty quickly.

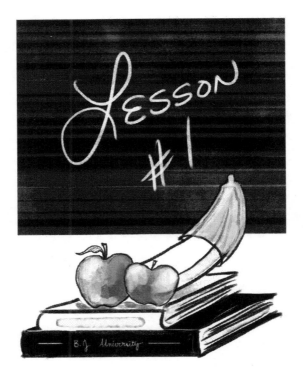

A month or so after my ex and I separated, a friend asked me if I wanted to take a class at a women's sex shop. The class was called BJ University. I always thought my skills in that particular area were decent, but a brushup certainly couldn't hurt! We made plans to have a quick dinner and a couple glasses of wine before going to the class (it seemed like it might be a little embarrassing without some "social lubrication"). Upon our arrival at the sex shop, we sat at tables with piles of dildos of all shapes and sizes, condoms, and lube in the center. There we were with about forty other nervous women, ready to be educated. And educated we became!

The first step was to choose a dildo, and I was very excited that I'd sprinted ahead of the rest of the group and gotten my hands on the biggest one. Until lesson number one: how to put a condom on with your mouth. The woman who taught the class (and owns the store) made it look pretty easy, but most of us needed a whole lot of practice to perfect the technique that she so masterfully demonstrated. I spent most of the time on that lesson gagging and wishing I'd chosen a more manageable size of dildo to work with.

The class continued with instructions on how to give ten— yes, ten—different types of blow jobs and hand jobs. We also learned about different types of lube and how to use it to make the "job" easier. I'd had no idea there were so many options! There we all were, stroking and sucking silicone cocks to the best of our abilities. I was in awe. I took notes. I still refer to them from time to time. And I've been told, by more than one fan, that that class was the best thirty-five dollars I've ever spent.

More and more sex shops for women are popping up around the country, so don't think you might not be able to find one! I highly recommend exploring them and asking anything that's on your mind. Really—they've heard it all, and are available to help you.

A side note: While visiting the sex shop, be sure to check out the lingerie. I find that most younger men *love* lingerie, and stores that specialize in the erotic arts are great places to find some really nice pieces for your wardrobe. I think wearing lovely bras and panties is one of the nicest things you can do for yourself—never mind that young men will appreciate it as well. Personally, it always adds a little spring in my step to know I've got something sexy going on, even under my work clothes and business suits!

Know Your Body, and Know Your Lube!

Lube, as I learned during my time at BJ University, is a complicated matter. The reason it's complicated is because there are so many options! While many of the options are a matter of personal taste, there are some general facts you should be aware of.

There are three families of lubricants: water-based, silicone-based, and oil-based. I'm here to tell you that research and my own experience have proven that oil-based lubes should never be used with latex condoms. Why: *The condoms will break,* and no one will be happy.

Silicone-based lubes are, in my experience, the best out there, because silicone is so easily absorbed into your body. Water-based lubes aren't bad, but you'll probably need to apply and reapply more frequently. Both make for an easy cleanup. (White 2014)

The stuff they sell in drugstores is OK in a pinch, but you have to be really careful about what you allow in your body in order for it to stay happy and healthy. Even the most resilient of bodies will rebel against certain chemicals, so be careful with scented lubricants and other unnatural ingredients.

Considering Condoms

Where lube is a choice, condoms are pretty much a necessity. I know, I know—sex feels a lot better without condoms, but unless and until you have a monogamous partner, you have to be safe. What I'm talking about in this book is about having fun, and fun **must** be responsible. Take care of yourself and your body (or you'll be in a perpetual state of STI panic)!

I haven't always been the queen of safe sex, especially at the beginning of my adventures as a single gal. Younger men seemed to think that they were being safe as long as they pulled out, and because I hadn't dealt with any of these for so many years, it all caught me a bit off guard. And, truth be told, I did go through an STI panic. A few times. But what really made me stick to my guns on safe sex was what happened with my twenty-eight-year-old friend Elizabeth.

Elizabeth, who I met at a hot yoga class, is a completely overeducated brainiac. She grew up in lily-white, upper-middle class, East Coast perfection. In college, she was on a committee that promoted safe sex and STI education. She never went anywhere without giving away condoms. There was no more perfect role model for safe and responsible sex than Elizabeth, the Preppy Condom Fairy.

So it came as a massive surprise when, at the juice bar after yoga one day, Elizabeth revealed to me that she'd had unprotected sex with a random guy that weekend. She was embarrassed that they hadn't used protection and had had no idea what'd gotten into her head, but we giggled about the escapade and then pretty much moved on.

Two weeks later, Elizabeth showed up to yoga, visibly upset. At the juice bar after class, Elizabeth told me that she'd heard from her random hookup from a few weeks before. To her horror, he told her he had just tested positive for HIV and Hepatitis C. Elizabeth cried in the juice bar, and I cried with her. She didn't know what to do. HIV has a certain incubation period, so she had to wait six weeks before she even got tested—and another two weeks for the test results. Fortunately, her test came back negative. Those nerve-racking two months of waiting, though, took a serious toll on both of us (we needed that yoga more than ever!), and neither of us have had unprotected sex since.

The good news (and Elizabeth agrees!) is that **this can all be prevented with condoms.** There are more options for condoms than you can count. Allergic to latex? Try polyure-thane, which is readily available at even your neighborhood Target. Vegan? Not to fret—there are vegan options too, and none of them break the bank! Like lube, condoms can come in varying flavors, which means you can be safe even during oral sex.

The nice thing is that companies that make condoms get that some people prefer the feel of unprotected sex. To that end, the many condom options cater to pleasure. There are ultra-thin condoms, ribbed condoms (for his AND her pleasure!), studded condoms, extra-lubricated condoms, and even silly ones that glow in the dark. **You. Have. Options.** There's no excuse! Protect yourself.

You can—and should—further protect yourself by not counting on men to provide condoms for you. Have your own stock. Guys will likely have cheaper varieties that might not do great things for your body. What's more, you can combat a potential argument of "I don't have a condom" by presenting one. Objections won't be easy if a condom is right in front of you! You might even bring up your commitment to safe sex before you meet. That way, you can lay down the ground rules so that you're ready to roll when the time comes.

Protection: Not Just for Private Parts

While I do believe that meeting online and checking out men before you meet them is safer than randomly meeting out somewhere, you do have to think about your personal safety. It should be common sense, but just in case it's not: Always, *always* meet in a public place. I usually suggest a bar that's convenient for me. A little liquid courage is absolutely fine when meeting someone new, and the lighting is usually good!

It's important to note here that you need to keep your wits about you. A first meeting rests heavily on your ability to listen to your gut instincts. Always trust yourself first and him, second. And—I can't stress this enough—watch your drink. Rohypnol (a.k.a. "roofies" and the "date-rape drug") isn't just an issue on college campuses! Even though the thirty-year-old consultant hottie checks out on LinkedIn, there's always the possibility that something is off.

If the two of you click and your eyes are locked and you start to feel nervous, like you're in a high-school romance, then fantastic! This type of chemistry is fun and exciting. This is what we're looking for. If you choose to go home with each other that evening, go for it. Again, I am not talking about meeting your husband here. I am talking about having fun. And sometimes you want to see how much fun you will be having sooner rather than later. **It's OK.** You are in control. You are making the decisions.

Eventually, you do end up at his place or your place (or maybe somewhere else entirely!). You've listened to your instincts and decided to take a chance with this guy. At this point, you do need to still err on the side of caution. It's terrible to think about, but you need to have an exit plan if something gets weird or doesn't feel right. If you're not in your own space, take just a second to look around for large objects that you can use in your defense if you need to. A little self-defense training isn't a bad idea either. I've never had any issues, but it's definitely something that you need to prepare yourself for. Verify his identity online, meet somewhere public, and listen to your intuition, but still have a plan to get yourself out of any situation. Preparedness is what helps you to stay in control!

Tales from Tinder: *Tony*

Tony was a thirty-one-year-old trader who was a real estate broker on the side. One evening, I mentioned that I was selling my condo where I'd lived with my ex and was looking for a new place to live. Tony immediately stepped up and helped me in my quest.

From that moment on, he was focused and all business! Moving out of what I thought was going to be my home for the rest of my life was ultimately very sad for me—but having a young, fun, *hot* real estate broker who picked me up and drove me around to apartment showings over the course of quite a few weekends was perfect. He set me up on MLS listings, arranged for all of the appointments, flirted with me, and treated me like a queen. What could have been a depressing process was suddenly fun and exciting. Ultimately, he did help me find an apartment that I fell in love with. I still live there—and we still stay in touch.

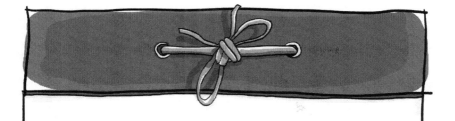

→ Investing in some sexy lingerie is one of the best—
and easiest—self-esteem boosters out there!

→ Don't forget to do your research! Taking an adult
sex-education class can bring you up to speed on
many modern sexual techniques and innovative
products that will greatly enhance your experience
in the bedroom.

→ Make certain to protect yourself from STIs by
always using condoms, as well as lubricants that
are best suited for the type of condom you choose.

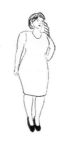

Chapter 5
Now Is Your Time

"What people seek is not the meaning of life,
but the experience of being alive."
— Joseph Campbell, American
mythologist, writer, and lecturer

As circumstance would have it, you are a single woman of a certain age. The scariest thing to me as I approached my divorce was the thought of dating again; I simply couldn't imagine it going well. It was challenging enough the first time around. How could I possibly endure the whole tedious process of going out, meeting men who actually wanted to talk to me, and dating again? Well, as you've seen, I was "alone" for a whole forty-eight hours! All of this is to say: It works out.

The game changes 100 percent when you're not looking for a husband. Suddenly, there's no checklist. Different men offer different things, and they're all interesting creatures. You learn to enjoy men for what they *do* have to offer, and to forget about everything else. There's no pressure—just the experience of meeting a new person. It doesn't matter, because you are in control. You are choosing what you want in your life.

What inspired me to write this book was, of course, the fantastic realization that many younger men adore older women—and my subsequent desire to shout this realization from the mountaintops! But the real point is that technology has enabled women to have the power to connect with any type of relationship they want, and that power is literally in the palm of their hands. This is something that women in their thirties, forties, fifties, and beyond naturally seek, deserve and should enjoy. And enjoying it really is what it's all about. Enjoying life, frankly, is what we all deserve!

Experience the World

Now is the time to live your life exactly the way you want to, and not just in the context of men. There's a new, fantastic world all around you, and there's no time like the present to explore it. Being single means being free. Use it.

A few months after my divorce was finalized, I got the travel bug. After binge-watching Anthony Bourdain's *No Reservations* all winter, it was time to make some plans. I decided that I'd

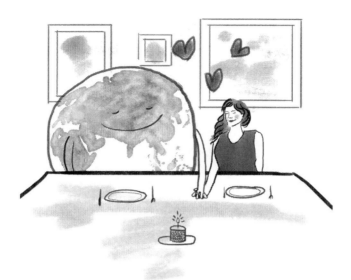

take a trip to celebrate my freedom and *my* life: five days in Paris followed by five days in London. I'd been to both cities before, but never alone. Now was the time.

There's nothing like putting yourself in a completely different environment (especially a different country and culture) to gain some perspective on whatever's going on in your life. Paris, the most romantic city in the world, actually held the key for me to escape the world of romance. It was magical. I didn't meet any men. It was Anne time. I'd wake up every day and go where I wanted to go. I ate when and what and where I wanted to eat. I took a nap if I felt like it. I went to a concert if I felt like it. I drank half a bottle of wine at a café if I felt like it. I bought expensive perfume if I felt like it. It was time for me.

It sounds indulgent, and maybe it was. What I was really doing, though, was taking very good care of myself. I stayed in an exclusive, quaint little hotel and reveled in it all. I understood that I was experiencing an astonishing sense of freedom, and I knew I owed it to myself to immerse myself in it and live it fully. I did just that, and I'm a better woman for it. I never could have done it or felt the beauty of the trip that completely if I'd been tied down. I needed to be 100 percent Anne to glean everything I could out of the new world around me.

Embrace Your Freedom

I'll be frank: I think being single is amazing. I love being able to do what I want to do, when I want to do it. That solo trip abroad made me realize that I'm in charge of my life, and I'm not beholden to anyone except myself anymore. If I don't want to cook dinner, I don't. If I don't want to make my bed, I don't. I bring that sense of freedom to my life, and I'm happy.

Rediscovering some simple pleasures has also been a part of my journey. What I love about adding simple pleasures to life is that it's easy to do, and each one brings richness—in a very big way—to an area where I previously had none at all. Here are some of my favorites to thrill and empower any single girl!

- Dine alone. Pick a restaurant that you love, find a little table in a spot that you're comfortable in, and just order a lovely meal and a glass of wine. Enjoy your meal. Become a regular at that restaurant, or at least make this simple thing a ritual in your life.

- Go to the movies alone on a Saturday morning! It's a great way to get yourself out of the house, and a movie may inspire your entire weekend. Plus, Saturday mornings are usually slow at the movies, which means you'll have a huge space to fully experience the movie you choose.

- Use your best dishes when you eat at home. Go ahead. Who's stopping you? Even if you're just heating up a frozen burrito, it'll make dining a lovely experience.

- Wear your best jewelry. Feeling pretty is such a simple thing, but it inspires us all to put our best feet forward. I have a pair of diamond studs that I adore, and they put me in touch with my own feelings of sophistication and confidence. I wear them every day!

- Keep learning. (Anything!) There are so many online courses, and podcasts and articles galore on any subject you can possibly imagine. Read up and give yourself some more perspective!

- Simplify your wardrobe. Prune that closet. If you haven't worn something in a year, give it a toss! Try on everything, and only keep what fits and what makes you look and feel your best.

Open Your Mind

Since my single journey through adulthood began, I've also become interested in energy, flow, and learning to operate in your "code," as my therapist would call it. Operating within your code means that you're doing things in your life that are natural to *you*. Those things may also give you a bit of a buzz; let them! They're things that make you light up and give you energy. Identifying those things and determining if you're doing enough of them is highly important to living a fulfilling life.

And on that note, why not see a therapist? So many of us do these days, but even if you don't feel like you have issues you really want to sort out, it's a great way to just get to know yourself a little better.

I've also been experimenting with some different energy therapies, such as Reiki and having my Akashic records opened. I've been quite skeptical of these kinds of therapies in the past, but I'm here to tell you that Reiki relaxed me, and my Akashic records pointed me in the direction of this book. Dive in! You never know what you'll find that opens you more to yourself.

Going through a big change in life—like divorce—allows a huge opportunity for reflection and spiritual exploration. Spirituality means a number of different things to a number of different people, but I think it comes down to knowing your soul and feeling the world around you. Change can propel you into certain understandings, and standing alone will give you the opportunity to head out in the direction in which you, yourself, deserve to go. It's your path, and it's your time. Find it. If you're looking for a little help in the relationship game, I'm here to help. Visit annegrey.com/consulting to schedule some 1:1 coaching time.

Tales from Tinder: *Arjun*

His name was Arjun. We matched, and right away he asked me out to dinner. No sexting, no requests for pictures, no asking my bra size (this does happen!). Arjun's profile said he was thirty-one and a consultant. That all worked for me—*and* he was polite and willing to reach out to me. I felt that something was going to be different here, and boy, was I right . . .

Dinner was lovely. Our conversation was fascinating. He loved looking into my light eyes, and I, into his dark. We connected, we held hands, we strolled through the city. We started seeing each other once a week. Then, twice a week. There were always dinners at which to connect at the end of our busy weeks, followed by the most fantastic sex that only improved the more we saw each other. I wasn't even officially divorced yet, but I was smitten. I loved seeing him. I grew to trust him. It was lovely. It was romantic. It grew for over three months. It blew my mind. This kind of thing wasn't supposed to happen on Tinder. I swiped right on him to get laid . . . and yet, here I was: in love.

As fate would have it, he ultimately had to move away to deal with a family issue. I was a bit heartbroken, but I understood—and really, I wasn't supposed to be having feelings for anyone at this point in my life anyway! So I let him go. (Not that there was an option to do otherwise.)

To this day, Arjun and I still see each other every few months for the most romantic, intense, passionate weekends I could ever imagine. Ever. Our time together is delicious, and it's everything that I have ever wanted. He treats me like a goddess, and I cherish my time in his arms and in his bed. As of the writing of this book, we are kept apart due to circumstance. There's nothing that I can do about this except put it out to the universe. If we're meant to be together, it will eventually work out. If not, we'll both be OK. I know from my experience with him that this is the type of relationship I want and deserve, with him or with someone else. Arjun is the gold standard, and I feel grateful for every minute we've had together.

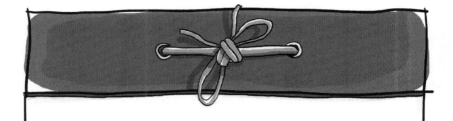

- → Technology has enabled women to have the power to connect with any type of relationship they want, and that power is literally in the palm of their hands!

- → From dining out on your own at elegant restaurants to exploring exciting new locales, it's important to rediscover some of the simple pleasures of being single.

- → Going through a big change in life—like divorce—allows a huge opportunity for reflection and spiritual exploration. It's your path and your time to explore exactly what makes you *you.*

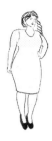

Chapter 6
We Are Made of Stars

Try this concept on for size: Everything and everyone are interconnected through energy. Think back to your high school physics class. If you're like me, you've probably tried to put that particular trauma out of your head entirely. *But,* there is one piece of information that I learned that has and will continue to stick with me, and it's called "The Law of Conservation of Energy."

It's pretty straightforward: Energy can be neither created nor destroyed. It just transforms and moves from one place to another. Have you ever played with a Newton's cradle? It's a line of hanging spheres, and when you pull the first one out and let it go, it hits the next one. That second sphere—and the third, and the fourth—stays still, but the sphere at the end of the chain bounces up. It's because the energy shoots through all of them and keeps going.

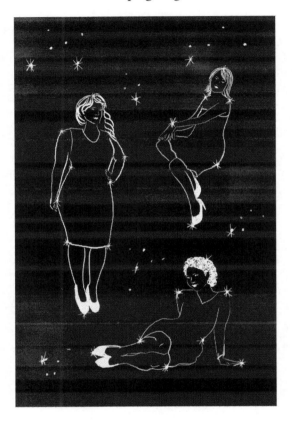

On a grander scale, that means that all of the energy in the universe is connected. The energy in your body, no doubt, contains a fragment of energy from an exploding star from millions of years ago. We're made of stars—we're related to everything that has ever existed. And that, my friends, means that your energy has the power to affect everyone else's energy.

As Dr. Christiane Northrup, expert in women's health and wellness, states, "Quantum physics" (the first law of which is what you just learned) "has proven beyond a doubt that all of us are interconnected energetically. So, when one woman awakens to the birthright of pleasure, she makes it that much easier for the next one to do the same . . . as a woman awakens sexually, she connects her intellect and her spirituality with her erotic anatomy, becoming a fully integrated force for good on the planet. So ring your bell and invite others to ring theirs!"

As I met up with friends and friends of friends over the last year to tell them about my journey, my hope was to inspire them to take the same risks that I did and reap the same rewards. But this idea that we're all connected energetically makes the idea so, so much more powerful. It's my hope that all women *everywhere* can embrace their sexuality, their needs, their desires, and their lives. That universal embracing begins with me, and it begins with you.

So rise to the challenge. Awaken to the control you have over who you want to have in your life and when. Awaken to the pleasure that you want and that you deserve. Awaken to the feminine power that you control. And enjoy it.

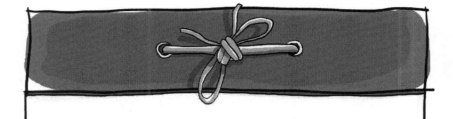

→ It's important to keep in mind that since everything and everyone are interconnected through energy, your personal energy has the power to affect the energy of those around you.

→ Remember to consistently embrace your needs, desires, sexuality, and individuality!

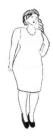

Conclusion

Well, dear reader, our time together is coming to an end. I hope that you've been able to find this book helpful, and you'll use it on your journey to the free-spirited, wild, crazy lust that we all deserve.

I'd like to stay in touch with you and hear of your own stories of dating, relationships, break-ups, love, love lost, Tinder, you name it! Please contribute these stories to:

www.annegrey.com

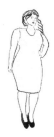

The Single Girl's Guide to Resources

1. Reaching Out

It seems like there are new dating apps popping up every day. The following are apps I have personally used and recommend, with summaries provided by Tom's Guide and POPSUGAR.

Tinder (Android, iOS)

Blazed the trail, set by Grindr, toward a new generation of swipe-and-scroll dating apps for the mobile set. In theory, you're not supposed to make shallow, snap judgments about potential partners, but Tinder encourages you to do just that.

You create a simple profile with a handful of photos and a few sentences about yourself, then throw yourself at the Internet's mercy. The app displays singles in your area. If you like one, swipe the photo to the right; otherwise, swipe to the left. If you and a match swipe right on each other, then you can send messages and set something up.

Coffee Meets Bagel (Android, iOS)

Aiming for quality over quantity, Coffee Meets Bagel (Android, iOS) brings you a single "bagel" every day: a curated match that shares mutual Facebook friends. You then have twenty-four hours to decide whether to like or to pass, with the app learning from your preferences. If you both express interest, CMB then brings you together in a private chat room, where you can get to know each other or plan a date. Other features, such as the ability to view your mutual friends, can be unlocked by purchasing a virtual currency called "beans."

Bumble (Android, iOS)

From the minds of previous Tinder executives comes Bumble, a newly released iOS app that lets women run the show. Like Tinder, Bumble lets users swipe right to approve and left to decline. If two users mutually swipe each other right, they are allowed to chat, but here's the kicker: Only women can initiate the conversation, and they only have twenty-four hours to do so before the connection disappears.

2. Feeling Good

The following is a pretty comprehensive list of the online and boutique retailers from which you can buy some very, very fun items. Don't hesitate to look for local stores too!

Adam & Eve www.adameve.com

Babeland www.babeland.com

Blowfish www.blowfish.com

Coco de Mer www.coco-de-mer.co.uk

Come as You Are www.comeasyouare.com

Early to Bed www.early2bed.com

Eros Boutique www.erosboutique.com

Eve's Garden www.evesgarden.com

Forbidden Fruit www.forbiddenfruit.com

G Boutique www.boutiqueg.com

Good for Her www.goodforher.com

Good Vibrations www.goodvibes.com

Grand Opening www.grandopening.com

JT's Stockroom www.stockroom.com

Libida www.libida.com

Liberator Shapes www.liberatorshapes.com

Pleasure Chest www.pleasurechest.com

Purple Passion www.purplepassion.com

Sh! www.sh-womenstore.com

Smitten Kitten www.smittenkittenonline.com

Vixen Creations www.vixencreations.com

Womyn's Ware www.womynsware.com

Xandria Collection www.xandria.com

3. Surfing the Net

These are some of my favorite websites to explore. They're great places to pick up some knowledge.

http://sexwithemily.com/

Leading sex expert and Bravo TV star Dr. Emily Morse offers the best sex tips, dating tips, and relationship advice that will change your love life today.

http://dodsonandross.com/

Betty Dodson and Carlin Ross are two intergenerational, sex-positive feminists whose dialogue on sexuality and feminism entertains and educates while delving into the politics of women's sexuality.

http://intimateartscenter.com/

We envision a world where sex is understood, honored, and free from shame, where our bodies' ecstatic potential is explored and celebrated, and relationships are based on integrity, compassion, and love.

http://puckerup.com/

Tristan Taormino's mission is to educate people of all genders and sexual orientations in their pursuit of healthy, empowering, and transformative sex and relationships. She spreads her pleasure-positive message through her books, films, writing, teaching, and lectures.

http://www.adiosbarbie.com/

Adiós, Barbie is the one-stop body-image shop for identity issues, including size, race, media, and more!

4. Read It

Big Magic: Creative Living Beyond Fear by Elizabeth Gilbert (Penguin 2015)

Come as You Are: The Surprising New Science that Will Transform Your Sex Life by Emily Nagoski, PhD (Simon & Schuster 2015)

Goddesses Never Age: The Secret Prescription for Radiance, Vitality, and Well-Being by Christiane Northrup, MD (Hay House, Inc. 2015)

Moody Bitches by Julie Holland, MD (Penguin 2015)

My Life on the Road by Gloria Steinem (Random House 2015)

Sex Outside the Lines: Authentic Sexuality in a Sexually Dysfunctional Culture by Chris Donaghue, PhD (BenBella Books 2015)

The Essential Rumi, New Expanded Edition by Jalal al-Din Rumi and Coleman Barks (HarperOne; Reprint Edition 2004)

5. Take a Listen

Death, Sex & Money

A podcast hosted by Anna Sale about the big questions and hard choices that are often left out of polite conversation.

Discover Your Inner Awesome

Listen to real conversations that help you kick ass at life. Learn how to better understand who you are, what you're doing, and where you're headed.

GUYS WE F**D: THE ANTI SLUT-SHAMING PODCAST**

They spread their legs, and now they're spreading the word that women should be able to have sex with WHOMEVER they want WHENEVER they want, and not be ashamed or called sluts or whores. Welcome to a new revolution.

HuffPost Love + Sex

A show that seeks to redefine the way we talk about love and sex by examining it from an anthropological perspective.

On Being

Krista Tippett takes up the big questions of meaning with scientists and theologians, artists and teachers—some you know and others you'll love to meet.

Only Human

A show about health that we all can relate to: "Because every body has a story."

Modern Love

Explore the trials and tribulations of love in these deeply personal essays.

Savage Lovecast

Love and sex advice from expert Dan Savage.

Strangers

Each episode is an empathy shot in your arm, featuring true stories about the people we meet, the connections we make, the heartbreaks we suffer, the kindnesses we encounter, and those frightful moments when we discover that WE aren't even who we thought we were.

Stuff Mom Never Told You

Hosted by Cristen Conger and Caroline Ervin, *Stuff Mom Never Told You* is the audio podcast from *HowStuffWorks* that gets down to the business of being women from every imaginable angle.

Unmistakable Creative

This is a collection of over five hundred interviews with thought leaders and people from all walks of life.

Women of the Hour

Lena Dunham hosts this podcast miniseries about friendship, love, work, bodies, and more.

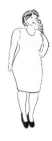

Bibliography

American, Scientific. "Sext Much? If So, You're Not Alone." *Scientific American.* February 4, 2014. http://www.scientificamerican.com/article/sext-much-if-so-youre-not-alone/ (accessed December 28, 2015).

Frezza, Bill. "Cheap Over-the-Counter STD Test Turbocharges Casual Sex." *Forbes Magazine.* October 22, 2013. http://www.forbes.com/sites/billfrezza/2013/10/22/cheap-over-the-counter-std-test-turbocharges-casual-sex/ (accessed December 28, 2015).

Kaiser, Frank. "In Praise of Older Women." *Suddenly Senior.* 01 01, 2000. www.suddenlysenior.com/praiseolderwomen.html (accessed 12 28, 2015).

Kaplan, Karen. "The Paradox of Millennial Sex." *LA Times.* May 9, 2015. http://www.latimes.com/science/sciencenow/la-sci-sn-millennials-sex-attitudes-20150508-story.html (accessed December 28, 2015).

Last, Walter. "The Neurochemistry of Sex." *Health Science Spirit.* December 28, 2015. http://www.health-science-spirit.com/neurosex.html (accessed December 28, 2015).

Popova, Maria. "When Woman is Boss." *Brain Pickings.* July 10, 2015. https://www.brainpickings.org/2015/07/10/nikola-tesla-when-woman-is-boss/ (accessed December 28, 2015).

Shpancer, Ph.D., Noam. "The Cougar Conundrum." *Psychology Today.* October 4, 2012. https://www.psychologytoday.com/blog/insight-therapy/201210/the-cougar-conundrum (accessed December 28, 2015).

SKYN. *SKYN Condoms Infographics.* December 28, 2015. http://us.skyncondoms.com/infographic/ (accessed December 28, 2015).

In Her Own Words. Directed by HBO Documentary Films Summer Series. Performed by Gloria Steinem. 2015.

Strgar, Wendy. "Healing Sex." *Making Love Sustainable.* May 29, 2015. http://makinglovesustainable.com/healing-sex-2/) (accessed December 28, 2015).

Tinder. "You Asked, We Listened: The Best Tinder Experiences." *Go Tinder.* November 11, 2015. http://blog.gotinder.com/ (accessed December 28, 2015).

Twenge, Jean M. "Changes in American Adults' Sexual Behavior and Attitudes, 1972-2002." *SpringerLink.* May 5, 2015. http://link.springer.com/article/10.1007/s10508-015-0540-2 (accessed December 28, 2015).

UTNews. "Ticking Biological Clock Increases Women's Libdo, New Research Shows." *UTNews.* July 7, 2010. http://news.utexas.edu/2010/07/07/psychology_biological_clock (accessed December 28, 2015).

Webb, Nadia. "The Neurobiology of Bliss." *Scientific American.* July 12, 2011. http://www.scientificamerican.com/article/the-neurobiology-of-bliss-sacred-and-profane/ (accessed December 28, 2015).

White, Melissa. "Wetter Is Better." *The Huffington Post.* January 14, 2014. http://www.huffingtonpost.com/melissa-white/wetter-is-better-how-to-choose-the-best-lube_b_4598397.html (accessed December 28, 2015).

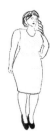

Acknowledgments

Thanks to my ex husband for leaving me.

Thanks to my friends who tolerated me.

Thanks to all the lovely men I met on Tinder.

And huge thanks to my therapist—seriously, she's amazing!

Notes Page

Dear Reader,

    This isn't homework! Think of it as a place for you to record your thoughts, either while you're reading, or as you're moving through your dating journey. Write down some fun memories; record things you like/don't like; take note of places you've been; etc!

Notes Page

53008571R00053

Made in the USA
San Bernardino, CA
11 September 2019